REAL FOOD FOR GESTATIONAL DIABETES

"Nourishing You and Your Baby: A Practical Guide to Managing Gestational Diabetes through Wholesome Nutrition"

EMMA LYNCH

EMMA LYNCH
Copyright © 2023 by [Emma Lynch]

TABLE OF CONTENTS

INTRODUCTION

Welcome to "Real Food for Gestational Diabetes: Nourishing You and Your Baby." This comprehensive guide is designed to empower expectant mothers facing the challenges of gestational diabetes with practical insights into managing their condition through a focus on wholesome nutrition.

Gestational diabetes, a form of diabetes that occurs during pregnancy, necessitates careful attention to dietary choices to maintain optimal health for both mother and baby. This guide aims to provide you with a roadmap for navigating this journey, offering valuable information, meal planning strategies, and a collection of delicious recipes centered around real, nutrient-dense foods.

In the following pages, we'll delve into the fundamentals of gestational diabetes, exploring its implications and the importance of adopting a diet rich in whole foods. From understanding carbohydrate management and balanced nutrition to incorporating lean proteins, whole grains, healthy fats, and a variety of fruits and vegetables, each section is crafted to offer practical guidance tailored to your unique needs.

We'll also provide creative snack ideas, a diverse recipe collection for every meal, and tips for making healthy choices when dining out. Recognizing the significance of physical activity during pregnancy, we've dedicated a section to safe exercise options. Additionally, we'll guide you through monitoring your blood sugar levels, offering insights into interpretation and tips for maintaining stable readings.

This guide is not just about managing gestational diabetes; it's about embracing a positive, proactive approach to your well-being and that of your growing baby. Connect with the support you need, whether it's through your healthcare providers, community resources, or further reading.

As you embark on this journey, remember that you have the ability to make informed choices that contribute to a healthy pregnancy. "Real Food for Gestational Diabetes" is here to guide you, providing a wealth of knowledge and practical tools to help you nourish both yourself and your baby, ensuring a positive and fulfilling pregnancy experience.

CHAPTER ONE

UNDERSTANDING GESTATIONAL DIABETES

Gestational diabetes is a specific type of diabetes that develops during pregnancy, typically around the second or third trimester. This condition is characterized by high blood sugar levels that, if not properly managed, can pose risks to both the mother and the baby. Understanding gestational diabetes involves exploring its causes, risk factors, effects on pregnancy, and the necessary measures for effective management.

Causes and Risk Factors:
Gestational diabetes occurs when the body is unable to produce enough insulin to meet the increased demands of pregnancy. One hormone that aids in controlling blood sugar levels is insulin. The placenta, which supports the baby's growth, produces hormones that can interfere with the mother's insulin function. As a result, glucose builds up in the bloodstream, leading to gestational diabetes.

Certain factors increase the risk of developing gestational diabetes, including being overweight before pregnancy, having a family history of diabetes, being older than 25, and belonging to certain ethnic groups. Additionally, women who have had gestational diabetes in a previous pregnancy are at an increased risk.

Effects on Pregnancy:
Gestational diabetes, if not properly managed, can have various effects on both the mother and the baby. For the mother, it may increase the risk of high blood pressure, preeclampsia, and the need for a cesarean section. It can also contribute to the development of type 2 diabetes later in life.

For the baby, gestational diabetes can lead to a condition known as macrosomia, where the baby grows larger than average. This increases the risk of birth injuries during delivery. Babies born to mothers with gestational diabetes may also experience low blood sugar levels (hypoglycemia) after birth.

Management and Monitoring:
Effective management of gestational diabetes involves a combination of lifestyle modifications, dietary changes, and, in some cases, medication. Regular monitoring of blood sugar levels is crucial, typically achieved through a combination of self-monitoring at home and periodic medical check-ups.

Dietary Considerations:
A key aspect of managing gestational diabetes is adopting a well-balanced diet. This includes

monitoring carbohydrate intake, choosing complex
carbohydrates over simple sugars, incorporating a
variety of nutrient-dense foods, and practicing
portion control. Nutritionists and healthcare
providers often play a vital role in helping pregnant
individuals plan meals that meet their specific
needs.

Physical Activity:
Regular, safe physical activity is encouraged as
part of gestational diabetes management. Exercise
helps lower blood sugar levels and can contribute
to overall well-being during pregnancy. However,
the type and intensity of exercise should be
discussed with healthcare providers to ensure
safety for both the mother and the baby.

Medical Support and Follow-up:
Regular prenatal check-ups are essential for
monitoring the progress of the pregnancy and the
well-being of both the mother and the baby.
Healthcare providers may recommend additional
ultrasounds and tests to assess the baby's growth
and well-being.

Postpartum Considerations:
After childbirth, blood sugar levels usually return to
normal. On the other hand, type 2 diabetes is more
likely to strike women who have experienced
gestational diabetes in the future. It's important to
continue healthy lifestyle practices, including

regular exercise and a balanced diet, and to undergo postpartum screening for diabetes.

In summary, understanding gestational diabetes involves recognizing its origins, appreciating its potential effects on pregnancy, and actively engaging in effective management strategies. To ensure a safe and successful pregnancy for themselves and their unborn children, women can manage gestational diabetes by collaborating closely with healthcare experts, embracing a healthy lifestyle, and following suggested monitoring and treatment regimens.

IMPORTANCE OF REAL FOOD

Real food, in its whole and unprocessed form, holds significant importance for overall health and well-being. Here are key aspects highlighting the importance of incorporating real food into one's diet:

1. **Nutrient Density:**
   Real foods, such as fruits, vegetables, whole grains, lean proteins, and healthy fats, are rich in essential nutrients like vitamins, minerals, antioxidants, and fiber. Nutrient-dense foods provide the body with the necessary building blocks for optimal functioning, supporting growth, energy production, and overall vitality.

2. **Balanced Nutrition:**
   Real foods offer a balanced combination of macronutrients (carbohydrates, proteins, and fats) and micronutrients (vitamins and minerals). This balance is essential for maintaining proper physiological functions, supporting immune health, and preventing nutritional deficiencies.

3. **Digestive Health:**
   Whole foods often contain dietary fiber, which plays a crucial role in digestive health. Constipation can be avoided, regular bowel movements are encouraged, and a healthy gut microbiota is supported by fiber. A well-functioning digestive system contributes to nutrient absorption and overall gut health.

4. **Blood Sugar Regulation:**
   Real foods, particularly those with complex carbohydrates and fiber, contribute to stable blood sugar levels. This helps prevent rapid spikes and crashes in blood sugar, reducing the risk of insulin resistance and type 2 diabetes.

5. **Satiety and Weight Management:**
   Generally speaking, whole foods satisfy better than processed foods. They provide a sense of fullness and satisfaction, which can contribute to better weight management by reducing overeating and snacking on empty-calorie foods.

6. **Heart Health:**
   Many real foods, such as fruits, vegetables, and nuts, are associated with cardiovascular health benefits. They contribute to lower blood pressure, reduced cholesterol levels, and a decreased risk of heart disease.

7. **Reduced Processed Additives:**
   Real foods are free from many of the additives, preservatives, and artificial ingredients often found in processed foods. By choosing real foods, individuals can reduce their exposure to potentially harmful substances and promote a more natural and wholesome diet.

8. **Mind-Body Connection:**
   A diet rich in real foods has been linked to improved mental health. Nutrient-dense foods provide essential nutrients that support cognitive function, mood regulation, and overall mental well-being.

9. **Disease Prevention:**
   Consuming a variety of real foods is associated with a lower risk of chronic diseases such as cardiovascular disease, certain cancers, and neurodegenerative conditions. Antioxidants present in many real foods play a role in protecting cells from damage.

10. **Environmental Impact:**

Choosing real foods often involves selecting fresh produce, whole grains, and sustainably sourced proteins. This can contribute to a more environmentally friendly and sustainable food system.

In essence, the importance of real food lies in its ability to nourish the body with essential nutrients, promote overall health, and reduce the risk of various health conditions. Making real food a fundamental part of one's diet supports long-term well-being and contributes to a healthier, more balanced lifestyle.

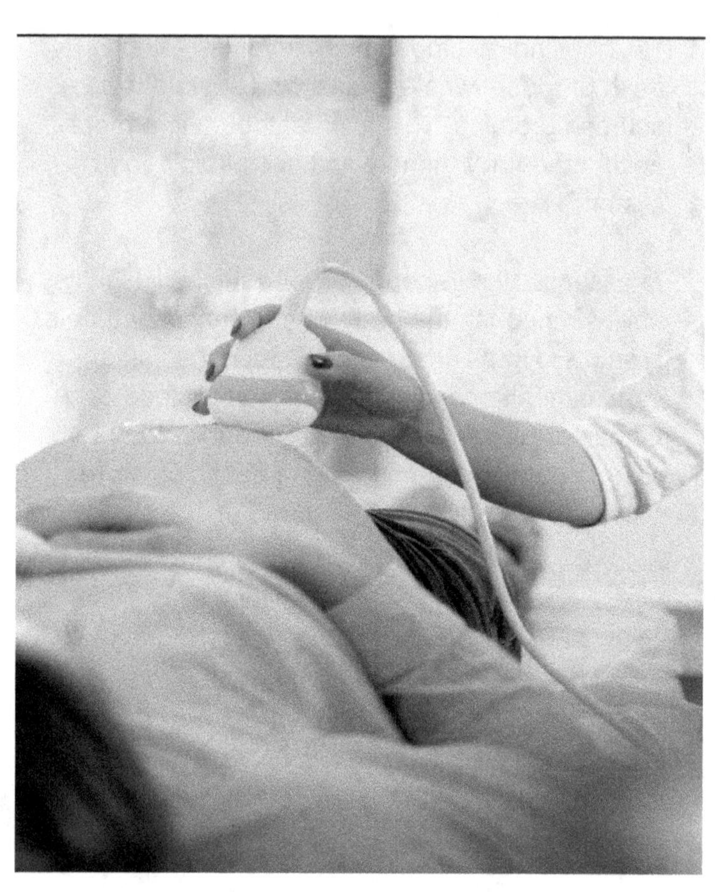

CHAPTER TWO

MEAL PLANNING

Meal planning is a valuable strategy for maintaining a balanced and nutritious diet. It involves thoughtfully organizing and preparing meals in advance, considering factors such as nutritional needs, taste preferences, and time constraints. Here's a guide to effective meal planning:

1. **Assess Nutritional Needs:**
   Identify your nutritional requirements based on factors like age, gender, activity level, and health goals. Consider any dietary restrictions or preferences.

2. **Create a Weekly Schedule:**
   Plan meals for the week, taking into account breakfast, lunch, dinner, and snacks. This helps ensure a balanced distribution of nutrients and prevents last-minute, less healthy food choices.

3. **Incorporate a Variety of Foods:**
   Aim for a diverse range of foods to ensure you get a spectrum of nutrients. Your meal plan should include whole grains, fruits, veggies, lean meats, and healthy fats.

4. **Portion Control:**

Take note of serving sizes to avoid overindulging. Use smaller plates, bowls, and utensils to help control portions and prevent excessive calorie intake.

5. **Preparation Time:**
Consider the time available for meal preparation on different days. Plan simpler recipes for busier days and reserve more complex meals for when you have additional time.

6. **Batch Cooking:**
Prepare larger quantities of meals and store leftovers for future use. This can save time and ensure you have convenient, healthy options readily available.

7. **Grocery Shopping:**
Create a shopping list based on your meal plan to streamline grocery shopping. Stick to your list to avoid impulsive purchases and ensure you have all the necessary ingredients.

8. **Seasonal and Local Produce:**
Consider incorporating seasonal and locally sourced produce into your meal plan. This not only supports local farmers but also ensures fresher, more flavorful ingredients.

9. **Mindful Snacking:**

Plan nutritious snacks to curb hunger between meals. Choose entire foods over processed snacks, such as nuts, fruits, and yogurt.

10. **Hydration:**
Don't forget about beverages. Include water as your primary beverage and consider incorporating herbal teas or infused water for variety.

11. **Flexibility:**
Allow for some flexibility in your meal plan to accommodate unexpected changes. Having a plan doesn't mean every meal must be rigidly followed.

12. **Try New Recipes:**
Keep meals interesting by incorporating new recipes into your plan. This can prevent boredom and increase the likelihood of sticking to your meal plan.

13. **Consider Dietary Preferences:**
Account for any specific dietary preferences or restrictions, such as vegetarian or gluten-free options, to ensure a satisfying and enjoyable eating experience.

14. **Family Considerations:**
If meal planning for a family, take into account the preferences and dietary needs of each family member. This can help create a harmonious and inclusive dining experience.

By investing time in thoughtful meal planning, you can make informed choices that align with your nutritional goals, save time during busy periods, and foster a healthier eating routine.

CARBOHYDRATE MANAGEMENT

Carbohydrate management is a crucial aspect of nutrition, particularly for individuals with conditions like diabetes, including gestational diabetes. This strategy involves controlling the intake and distribution of carbohydrates to regulate blood sugar levels. Here's a detailed explanation of carbohydrate management:

1. **Understanding Carbohydrates:**
   Carbohydrates are one of the three main macronutrients, along with proteins and fats. They are the main energy source for the body. Carbohydrates include sugars, starches, and fiber, and they are found in various foods such as grains, fruits, vegetables, legumes, and dairy products.

2. **Effect on Blood Sugar:**
   When consumed, carbohydrates are broken down into glucose (sugar), which enters the bloodstream. In individuals with diabetes or gestational diabetes, the body may struggle to produce enough insulin or use it effectively, leading to elevated blood sugar levels.

3. **Glycemic Index (GI):**
   The rate at which a food high in carbohydrates raises blood sugar is measured by the glycemic index. Blood sugar rises more slowly and gradually in response to foods with a low GI than in response to those with a high GI. Managing carbohydrate intake often involves choosing foods with a lower glycemic index.

4. **Carbohydrate Counting:**
   Carbohydrate counting is a common method used in carbohydrate management. It involves tracking the total grams of carbohydrates consumed in a meal or snack. This practice helps individuals with diabetes match their insulin doses to the amount of carbohydrates they eat.

5. **Meal Planning:**
   When managing carbohydrates, it's important to distribute them evenly throughout the day. This helps maintain stable blood sugar levels and prevents large spikes or crashes. Including a balance of carbohydrates, proteins, and fats in each meal contributes to sustained energy.

6. **Types of Carbohydrates:**
   The effects of various carbs on blood sugar vary. Simple carbohydrates, found in sugary foods and refined grains, tend to cause rapid spikes. Complex carbohydrates, found in whole grains, fruits, and vegetables, are absorbed more slowly, providing a steadier source of energy.

7. **Fiber Content:**
Including high-fiber foods is beneficial for carbohydrate management. Fiber slows down the digestion and absorption of carbohydrates, helping to control blood sugar levels. Legumes, whole grains, fruits, and vegetables are all excellent providers of fiber.

8. **Monitoring Blood Sugar Levels:**
Regular monitoring of blood sugar levels is crucial for effective carbohydrate management. This allows individuals to understand how different foods and meals impact their blood sugar and make necessary adjustments to their dietary choices or insulin doses.

9. **Individualized Approach:**
Carbohydrate management is highly individualized. Factors such as age, activity level, medications, and overall health impact the body's response to carbohydrates. Working with healthcare providers or registered dietitians is essential to tailor carbohydrate management strategies to individual needs.

10. **Education and Support:**
Education plays a key role in successful carbohydrate management. Individuals benefit from understanding the nutritional content of foods, how to read food labels, and the principles of carbohydrate counting. Support from healthcare

professionals, nutritionists, or diabetes educators is valuable in this process.

11. **Consistency and Flexibility:**
   Consistency in carbohydrate intake is important, but flexibility is also key. Individuals should be able to adapt their carbohydrate management to different situations, such as special occasions or changes in routine, while still maintaining blood sugar control.

12. **Lifestyle Factors:**
   Lifestyle factors, including regular physical activity, also influence carbohydrate management. The body can utilise glucose more effectively with improved insulin sensitivity brought on by exercise. Coordination between carbohydrate intake and exercise is crucial for maintaining blood sugar balance.

In summary, carbohydrate management involves making informed choices about the types and amounts of carbohydrates consumed to regulate blood sugar levels. This strategy is integral for individuals with diabetes or gestational diabetes and requires a personalized, well-rounded approach that considers various factors impacting individual health and well-being. Working collaboratively with healthcare professionals ensures a comprehensive and effective carbohydrate management plan.

BALANCED NUTRITION

Balanced nutrition is essential for managing gestational diabetes, ensuring both maternal health and the optimal development of the baby. Here's a detailed explanation of balanced nutrition specifically tailored to real food for gestational diabetes:

1. **Carbohydrate Management:**
   - Give priority to complex carbs that have a low glycemic index, like non-starchy vegetables, legumes, and whole grains.
   - Distribute carbohydrate intake evenly throughout the day to prevent large spikes in blood sugar levels.
   - Be mindful of portion sizes, and consider carbohydrate counting as a strategy for managing blood sugar.

2. **Lean Proteins:**
   - Include lean protein sources in every meal to help stabilize blood sugar levels and support fetal development.
   - Options include poultry, fish, lean meats, tofu, legumes, and low-fat dairy.

3. **Healthy Fats:**
   - Incorporate sources of healthy fats, such as avocados, nuts, seeds, and olive oil, into your meals.

- Healthy fats play a role in fetal brain development and contribute to satiety.

4. **Fiber-Rich Foods:**
   - Choose high-fiber foods like whole grains, fruits, vegetables, and legumes to support digestion and regulate blood sugar levels.
   - Additionally, fiber helps one feel fuller, which discourages overeating.

5. **Vitamins and Minerals:**
   - Ensure a diverse intake of fruits and vegetables to provide essential vitamins and minerals.
   - These nutrients are crucial for both maternal health and fetal development.

6. **Balanced Meal Composition:**
   - Adopt a balanced plate composition with half the plate filled with non-starchy vegetables, a quarter with lean protein, and a quarter with whole grains or starchy vegetables.
   - This approach ensures a variety of nutrients in each meal.

7. **Hydration:**
   - Sip plenty of water to stay well-hydrated during the day. Proper hydration supports overall health and can help regulate blood sugar levels.
   - Limit your intake of sugary and caffeinated beverages.

8. **Limiting Added Sugars:**

- Minimize the consumption of foods and beverages with added sugars. Opt for naturally sweet options like fruits to satisfy cravings.
  - Monitor food labels for hidden sugars in processed foods.

9. **Meal Timing:**
  - Maintain a consistent meal schedule, spacing meals evenly throughout the day to regulate blood sugar levels.
  - Include healthy snacks between meals to prevent excessive hunger.

10. **Individualized Approach:**
  - Work with healthcare providers, including registered dietitians, to create an individualized nutrition plan based on specific needs, health goals, and blood sugar monitoring results.
  - Adjustments may be necessary throughout pregnancy.

11. **Physical Activity:**
  - Incorporate safe and regular physical activity into your routine, as exercise helps manage blood sugar levels.
  - Choose activities that align with your fitness level and consult with healthcare providers for guidance.

12. **Stress Management:**

- Practice stress-reducing techniques, such as mindfulness, meditation, or gentle exercises like prenatal yoga.
    - High stress levels can impact blood sugar levels, and managing stress is vital during pregnancy.

13. **Regular Monitoring:**
    - Regularly monitor blood sugar levels as recommended by healthcare providers. This information guides adjustments to dietary choices, portion sizes, and overall management.

14. **Educational Resources:**
    - Utilize educational resources provided by healthcare professionals to enhance your understanding of gestational diabetes management.
    - Stay informed about the principles of balanced nutrition, portion control, and the impact of different food choices.

15. **Listening to Body Signals:**
    - Recognize when your body sends signals to you to feel hungry or full. Eating slowly and mindfully can prevent overeating and promote a healthy relationship with food.

By adopting a real food approach and focusing on balanced nutrition, individuals with gestational diabetes can support their health and the well-being of their babies. Customizing dietary choices to individual needs, monitoring blood sugar levels, and collaborating with healthcare professionals contribute to a successful and healthy pregnancy journey.

PORTION CONTROL

Portion control is particularly crucial for individuals with gestational diabetes, as it helps manage blood sugar levels and ensures a balanced intake of nutrients. Here's a detailed explanation of portion control tailored to real food for gestational diabetes:

1. **Understanding Carbohydrates:**
   Given the impact of carbohydrates on blood sugar levels, portion control becomes especially important for individuals with gestational diabetes. Focus on controlling portions of carbohydrates, considering both the type and quantity.

2. **Carbohydrate Counting:**
   Learn to count carbohydrates to manage blood sugar effectively. This involves understanding the carbohydrate content of different foods, reading nutrition labels, and keeping track of daily carbohydrate intake to distribute it evenly across meals and snacks.

3. **Balancing Nutrients:**
   Ensure a balanced intake of carbohydrates, proteins, and fats in each meal. This helps stabilize blood sugar levels and provides a steady source of energy. Include a variety of real foods such as lean

proteins, whole grains, fruits, vegetables, and healthy fats.

4. **Choose Whole Foods:**
   Choose nutrient-dense, whole, minimally processed foods. Whole grains, lean proteins, and high-fiber fruits and vegetables are excellent choices. These foods not only provide essential nutrients but also contribute to prolonged feelings of fullness.

5. **Plate Method:**
   To illustrate portion control, apply the plate method. Arrange your plate such that non-starchy vegetables make up half of it, lean protein makes up quarter of it, and whole grains or starchy veggies make up the other quarter. This approach ensures a balanced and diabetes-friendly meal.

6. **Smaller, Frequent Meals:**
   Think about eating more often and in smaller portions throughout the day. This can help prevent large spikes in blood sugar levels and keep them more stable.

7. **Portion Size Guidelines:**
   Familiarize yourself with portion size guidelines for different food groups. For example, a serving of lean protein might be about the size of a deck of cards, a serving of cooked grains the size of a tennis ball, and a serving of fruit the size of a small fist.

8. **Smart Snacking:**
   Plan snacks that are both satisfying and
diabetes-friendly. Combine protein with a small
amount of healthy fats or fiber to help stabilize
blood sugar levels between meals.

9. **Hydration:**
   Stay hydrated with water throughout the day.
Sometimes, feelings of hunger can be mistaken for
thirst. Drink less sugary drinks and more water or
herbal teas.

10. **Food Diary:**
   Keep a food diary to track your meals, snacks,
and blood sugar levels. This can help identify
patterns, trigger foods, and understand how
different portions affect your blood sugar.

11. **Meal Timing:**
   Stick to a regular eating schedule. Timing meals
consistently can help control blood sugar levels and
avoid sharp swings.

12. **Individualized Approach:**
   Work with your healthcare team or a registered
dietitian to develop an individualized portion control
plan. They can provide personalized guidance
based on your specific nutritional needs, health
goals, and lifestyle.

13. **Meal Preparation:**

Plan and prepare meals in advance to avoid spontaneous, potentially less healthy choices. Having appropriately portioned, diabetes-friendly meals readily available can simplify the process of adhering to portion control.

14. **Support System:**
Engage with a support system that includes healthcare professionals, family, and friends. Having a network that understands the importance of portion control for gestational diabetes can provide encouragement and practical assistance.

15. **Flexibility and Self-Compassion:**
Recognize that gestational diabetes management may require adjustments, and be flexible with your approach. Allow yourself some flexibility while staying committed to making healthy choices and practicing portion control.

By incorporating these strategies into daily life, individuals with gestational diabetes can effectively manage their blood sugar levels through portion control while enjoying a variety of real, nutrient-dense foods that assist the mother's and the child's health.

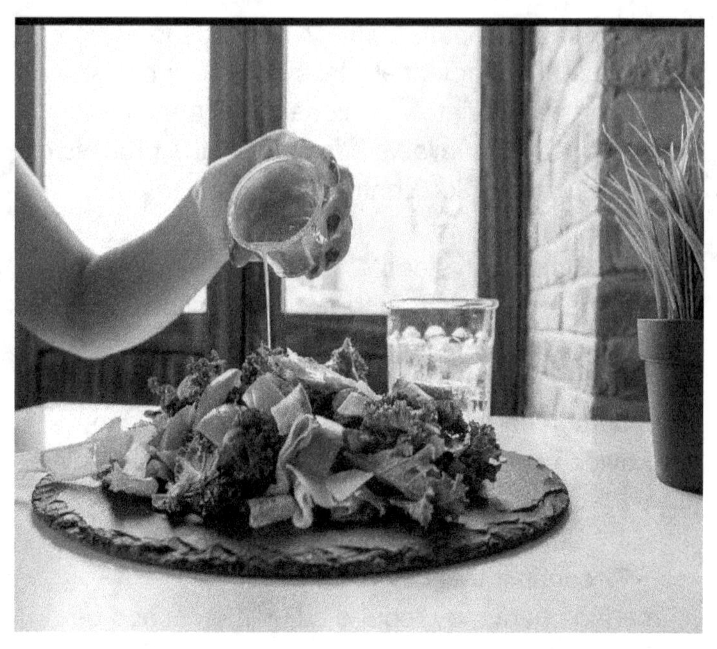

CHAPTER THREE

REAL FOOD OPTIONS

Real food options for gestational diabetes involve choosing nutrient-dense, minimally processed foods that support blood sugar management and provide essential nutrients for both the mother and the baby. Here's a detailed explanation:

1. **Non-Starchy Vegetables:**
   - Incorporate a range of non-starchy veggies, including bell peppers, zucchini, broccoli, cauliflower, and leafy greens.
   - These vegetables are high in fiber, vitamins, and minerals without causing significant spikes in blood sugar.

2. **Whole Grains:**
   - Opt for whole grains like quinoa, brown rice, barley, and oats instead of refined grains.
   - Whole grains provide fiber, essential nutrients, and a slower release of glucose, helping to regulate blood sugar levels.

3. **Lean Proteins:**
   - Choose lean protein sources to support muscle health and stabilize blood sugar. Options include poultry, fish, lean meats, tofu, and legumes.

- Protein-rich foods contribute to a feeling of fullness and help manage post-meal blood sugar levels.

4. **Healthy Fats:**
   - Include foods high in healthful fats, like olive oil, avocados, nuts, and seeds.
   - Healthy fats support fetal brain development, contribute to satiety, and can help manage blood sugar.

5. **Dairy or Dairy Alternatives:**
   - Include low-fat or non-fat dairy products or fortified dairy alternatives to meet calcium and vitamin D needs.
   - Choose options without added sugars to support overall health.

6. **Fruits in Moderation:**
   - Enjoy fruits in moderation, focusing on those with lower glycemic index values such as berries, cherries, and apples.
   - Pair fruits with protein or healthy fats to mitigate their impact on blood sugar levels.

7. **Nuts and Seeds:**
   - Snack on nuts and seeds like almonds, walnuts, chia seeds, or flaxseeds for healthy fats, protein, and fiber.
   - These options provide sustained energy and can help manage hunger between meals.

8. **Legumes:**
   - Incorporate legumes such as lentils, chickpeas, and black beans for plant-based protein, fiber, and a gradual release of glucose.
   - Legumes contribute to satiety and support digestive health.

9. **Eggs:**
   - Eggs are a nutrient-dense protein source and a versatile ingredient in various dishes.
   - They provide essential nutrients like choline, which is important for fetal brain development.

10. **Fish Rich in Omega-3 Fatty Acids:**
    - Choose fatty fish like salmon, mackerel, or trout, rich in omega-3 fatty acids.
    - Omega-3s support fetal brain and eye development and have potential benefits for blood sugar regulation.

11. **Natural Sweeteners in Moderation:**
    - Use natural sweeteners like stevia or monk fruit in moderation to sweeten foods or beverages.
    - Be cautious with the overall intake of sweeteners to avoid unnecessary spikes in blood sugar.

12. **Herbs and Spices:**
    - Enhance the flavor of meals with herbs and spices like cinnamon, turmeric, and ginger.
    - Some herbs and spices may have potential benefits for blood sugar regulation.

13. **Hydration with Water:**
   - Sip plenty of water to stay well-hydrated during the day.
   - Limit sugary beverages and caffeinated drinks, opting for water as the primary beverage.

14. **Meal Planning and Preparation:**
   - Plan and prepare meals in advance, focusing on a balance of nutrient-dense foods.
   - Batch cooking can be helpful for having wholesome options readily available.

15. **Portion Control:**
   - Practice portion control to manage overall caloric intake and prevent overeating.
   - Be mindful of carbohydrate portions and distribute them evenly throughout the day.

16. **Regular Monitoring:**
   - Regularly monitor blood sugar levels to understand how different real food options affect your body.
   - Use this information to make informed choices and adjust your meal plan as needed.

17. **Consultation with Healthcare Professionals:**
   - Work closely with healthcare providers, including registered dietitians, to tailor real food choices to your specific needs and monitor overall health throughout pregnancy.

By prioritizing these real food options, individuals with gestational diabetes can create a balanced and nourishing meal plan that supports blood sugar management, promotes overall health, and contributes to a healthy pregnancy.

LEAN PROTEIN

Lean protein is a crucial component of a well-balanced diet for individuals with gestational diabetes. It provides essential nutrients, supports fetal development, and helps manage blood sugar levels. Here's a detailed explanation of lean protein for gestational diabetes:

1. **Importance of Lean Protein:**
   - Lean protein is a valuable source of high-quality protein without excessive saturated fats.
   - Protein is essential for the development of the baby's organs, muscles, and tissues during pregnancy.

2. **Sources of Lean Protein:**
   - Choose lean protein sources that are lower in saturated fats. Examples include:
      - Poultry: Skinless chicken or turkey.
      - Fish: Omega-3 fatty acids are abundant in fatty fish, including trout, sardines, and salmon.
      - Lean Meats: Opt for lean cuts of beef or pork, trimming visible fat.

- Plant-Based Proteins: Tofu, tempeh, legumes (beans and lentils), and edamame are excellent vegetarian options.

3. **Eggs:**
   - Eggs are a flexible and high-nutrient protein source.
   - They provide essential nutrients, including choline, which is crucial for fetal brain development.

4. **Portion Control:**
   - Practice portion control to avoid excessive calorie intake while ensuring an adequate protein intake.
   - Aim for a serving size that aligns with your individual dietary needs and gestational stage.

5. **Meal Distribution:**
   - Distribute protein intake evenly throughout the day, including it in each meal and snack.
   - This helps maintain steady blood sugar levels and provides a consistent source of amino acids for the baby's development.

6. **Cooking Methods:**
   - Choose healthier cooking methods such as grilling, baking, broiling, or steaming to retain the nutritional value of lean proteins.
   - Minimize frying or cooking with excessive oils.

7. **Pairing with Fiber-Rich Foods:**

- Combine lean protein with high-fiber foods like vegetables, whole grains, and legumes.
- This pairing helps regulate blood sugar levels and promotes a feeling of fullness.

8. **Avoiding Processed Meats:**
- Limit or avoid processed meats such as sausages, hot dogs, and deli meats that may contain additives and higher levels of sodium.
- Choose fresh, unprocessed options whenever possible.

9. **Monitoring Blood Sugar Levels:**
- Regularly monitor blood sugar levels to understand how different protein sources affect your body.
- Adjust protein intake as needed to maintain stable blood sugar levels.

10. **Hydration:**
- Sip water to stay hydrated throughout the day.
- Adequate hydration supports overall health and can aid in digestion.

11. **Consultation with Healthcare Providers:**
- Consult with healthcare providers, including registered dietitians and obstetricians, to determine individual protein needs based on factors like weight, activity level, and overall health.

12. **Variety in Protein Sources:**

- Include a variety of lean protein sources in your diet to ensure a broad spectrum of essential amino acids and nutrients.
- This variety also prevents dietary monotony and enhances overall nutritional intake.

13. **Individualized Approach:**
- Customize your protein intake based on individual preferences, dietary restrictions, and cultural considerations.
- Tailoring your diet to your unique needs enhances adherence to a healthy eating plan.

14. **Supplementation if Needed:**
- If dietary intake is inadequate, medical professionals may occasionally suggest protein supplements.
- Discuss any supplementation with your healthcare team to ensure it aligns with your specific needs.

15. **Meal Planning and Preparation:**
- Plan and prepare meals in advance, incorporating a variety of lean protein sources to create well-balanced and satisfying dishes.

By incorporating lean protein into a well-rounded diet, individuals with gestational diabetes can meet their nutritional needs, support fetal development, and manage blood sugar levels effectively. A personalized approach, regular monitoring, and

collaboration with healthcare professionals
contribute to a healthy and successful pregnancy.

WHOLE GRAINS

Whole grains are an essential component of a
balanced diet for individuals with gestational
diabetes. They provide important nutrients, dietary
fiber, and a gradual release of glucose, helping to
manage blood sugar levels. Here's a detailed
explanation of whole grains for gestational
diabetes:

1. **Nutrient Density:**
   - Whole grains, such as brown rice, quinoa, oats,
and whole wheat, are rich in essential nutrients like
fiber, vitamins, and minerals.
   - These nutrients support overall health, including
fetal development and maternal well-being.

2. **Dietary Fiber:**
   - The high fiber content in whole grains
contributes to improved digestion and helps
regulate blood sugar levels.
   - Fiber slows down the absorption of glucose,
preventing rapid spikes and promoting a more
stable glycemic response.

3. **Complex Carbohydrates:**

- Whole grains contain complex carbohydrates, offering a sustained release of energy compared to refined grains.
  - This sustained energy can help prevent excessive hunger and support steady blood sugar levels.

4. **Stabilizing Blood Sugar Levels:**
  - The fiber and complex carbohydrates in whole grains contribute to better blood sugar control, making them a suitable choice for individuals with gestational diabetes.

5. **Variety of Whole Grains:**
  - Include a variety of whole grains in your diet to ensure a diverse range of nutrients. Examples include quinoa, barley, bulgur, farro, and whole grain pasta.
  - Experimenting with different whole grains adds variety to meals and prevents dietary monotony.

6. **Portion Control:**
  - Practice portion control when incorporating whole grains into your meals to manage overall carbohydrate intake.
  - Be mindful of serving sizes to avoid excessive caloric consumption.

7. **Meal Timing:**
  - Distribute whole grain intake evenly throughout the day, incorporating them into meals and snacks.

- This helps maintain a consistent supply of nutrients and supports blood sugar stability.

8. **Cooking Methods:**
   - Choose healthier cooking methods such as steaming, boiling, or baking to retain the nutritional value of whole grains.
   - Avoid excessive use of added fats or sugars in preparation.

9. **Whole Grain Breakfast Options:**
   - Opt for whole grain options in breakfast foods such as oatmeal, whole grain cereal, or whole grain toast.
   - Pairing whole grains with protein-rich foods can create a satisfying and balanced meal.

10. **Whole Grain Snacks:**
    - Choose whole grain snacks, such as whole grain crackers, popcorn, or whole grain granola bars.
    - Pairing these snacks with a source of protein can help manage blood sugar levels between meals.

11. **Reading Labels:**
    - When selecting packaged products, read labels carefully to ensure they contain whole grains as a primary ingredient.
    - Look for phrases in the ingredient list like "whole wheat" or "whole grain".

12. **Hydration:**
   - Stay well-hydrated by sipping water throughout the day, supporting overall health and digestion.
   - Restrict your intake of sugary and caffeinated beverages.

13. **Consultation with Healthcare Providers:**
   - Consult with healthcare providers, including registered dietitians, to determine individual carbohydrate needs and incorporate whole grains appropriately.

14. **Educational Resources:**
   - Utilize educational resources provided by healthcare professionals to enhance your understanding of gestational diabetes management, including the role of whole grains.

15. **Individualized Approach:**
   - Customize your whole grain choices based on personal preferences, cultural considerations, and any dietary restrictions.
   - An individualized approach enhances adherence to a healthy eating plan.

16. **Meal Planning and Preparation:**
   - Plan and prepare meals in advance, incorporating a variety of whole grains to create nourishing and well-balanced dishes.

By prioritizing whole grains in the diet, individuals with gestational diabetes can enjoy a wide range of nutrients while managing blood sugar levels effectively. Customizing dietary choices, practicing portion control, and collaborating with healthcare professionals contribute to a healthy and successful pregnancy.

HEALTHY FATS

Incorporating healthy fats into the diet is crucial for individuals with gestational diabetes, as they play a vital role in supporting overall health, fetal development, and blood sugar management. Here's a detailed explanation of healthy fats for gestational diabetes:

1. **Importance of Healthy Fats:**
   - A baby's brain and nervous system growth depends on healthy fats.
   - They also contribute to hormone production, absorption of fat-soluble vitamins (A, D, E, K), and overall cellular function.

2. **Sources of Healthy Fats:**
   - Include a variety of sources of healthy fats in your diet, such as:
     - Avocados: Rich in monounsaturated fats and provide essential nutrients.
     - Nuts and Seeds: Good sources of good fats include flaxseeds, chia seeds, walnuts, and almonds.
     - Olive Oil: Extra virgin olive oil is a heart-healthy option with monounsaturated fats.

- Fatty Fish: Salmon, mackerel, and trout contain omega-3 fatty acids, crucial for fetal development.

3. **Omega-3 Fatty Acids:**
   - Fatty fish and certain plant-based sources, like chia seeds and flaxseeds, contain omega-3 fatty acids.
   - Omega-3s support fetal brain and eye development and may have potential benefits for blood sugar regulation.

4. **Monounsaturated Fats:**
   - Foods high in monounsaturated fats, such as avocados and olive oil, are excellent choices.
   - Monounsaturated fats are known for their heart-healthy properties and can be part of a balanced diet.

5. **Polyunsaturated Fats:**
   - Polyunsaturated fats, found in nuts, seeds, and certain oils, provide essential fatty acids that the body cannot produce on its own.
   - They contribute to overall health and should be included in moderation.

6. **Coconut Oil and Saturated Fats:**
   - While coconut oil contains saturated fats, it can be included in moderation.
   - However, it's important to balance saturated fat intake with other healthy fat sources.

7. **Portion Control:**
   - Practice portion control when incorporating healthy fats into meals and snacks to manage overall calorie intake.
   - Pay attention to portion proportions to prevent overindulging.

8. **Cooking Methods:**
   - Choose healthier cooking methods that preserve the nutritional value of healthy fats.
   - Options include using olive oil for sautéing, incorporating avocados into salads, and incorporating nuts and seeds into meals.

9. **Adding Healthy Fats to Meals:**
   - Enhance the nutritional profile of meals by adding sliced avocado to salads, sprinkling nuts or seeds on yogurt, or drizzling olive oil on vegetables.
   - These additions contribute flavor and texture while providing essential nutrients.

10. **Consultation with Healthcare Providers:**
   - Consult with healthcare providers, including registered dietitians, to determine individual dietary needs and incorporate healthy fats appropriately.

11. **Educational Resources:**
   - Utilize educational resources provided by healthcare professionals to enhance your understanding of gestational diabetes management, including the role of healthy fats.

12. **Individualized Approach:**
   - Customize your choices of healthy fats based on personal preferences, cultural considerations, and any dietary restrictions.
   - An individualized approach enhances adherence to a healthy eating plan.

13. **Meal Planning and Preparation:**
   - Plan and prepare meals in advance, incorporating a variety of healthy fats to create flavorful and well-balanced dishes.

By prioritizing healthy fats in the diet, individuals with gestational diabetes can support their overall health, fetal development, and blood sugar management. A balanced approach, portion control, and collaboration with healthcare professionals contribute to a healthy and successful pregnancy.

FRUITS AND VEGETABLES

Incorporating a variety of fruits and vegetables into the diet is essential for individuals with gestational diabetes. These nutrient-dense foods provide essential vitamins, minerals, fiber, and antioxidants while supporting blood sugar management. Here's a detailed explanation of fruits and vegetables for gestational diabetes:

1. **Nutrient Density:**

- Fruits and vegetables are rich in essential nutrients, including vitamins, minerals, and antioxidants.
   - Nutrient-dense choices support overall health, including fetal development and maternal well-being.

2. **Fiber Content:**
   - High fiber content in fruits and vegetables aids in digestion and helps regulate blood sugar levels.
   - Fiber slows down the absorption of glucose, preventing rapid spikes and promoting a more stable glycemic response.

3. **Low Glycemic Index Options:**
   - Choose fruits and vegetables with a low glycemic index to minimize their impact on blood sugar levels.
   - Examples of low-GI options include berries, cherries, leafy greens, and non-starchy vegetables.

4. **Variety of Colors and Types:**
   - Include a variety of colorful fruits and vegetables to ensure a diverse range of nutrients.
   - Different colors often indicate various phytonutrients, each with unique health benefits.

5. **Non-Starchy Vegetables:**
   - Leafy greens, broccoli, cauliflower, and bell peppers are good examples of non-starchy veggies.

- They are low in carbohydrates and calories while providing essential vitamins and minerals.

6. **Starchy Vegetables in Moderation:**
   - Include starchy vegetables like sweet potatoes, carrots, and peas in moderation.
   - Pairing them with protein or healthy fats can help manage their impact on blood sugar levels.

7. **Fruits in Moderation:**
   - Enjoy fruits in moderation, focusing on those with lower glycemic index values, such as berries, cherries, and apples.
   - Pairing fruits with protein or healthy fats can help mitigate their impact on blood sugar levels.

8. **Whole Fruits vs. Juices:**
   - Choose whole fruits over fruit juices to benefit from the fiber content and slow the absorption of sugars.
   - Limit fruit juice intake due to its concentrated sugar content.

9. **Portion Control:**
   - Practice portion control when incorporating fruits and vegetables into meals and snacks.
   - Be mindful of overall carbohydrate intake to manage blood sugar levels effectively.

10. **Cooking Methods:**

- Opt for healthier cooking methods like steaming, roasting, or sautéing to preserve the nutritional value of fruits and vegetables.
   - Minimize the use of added fats or sugars in preparation.

11. **Adding Vegetables to Meals:**
   - Enhance the nutritional profile of meals by adding a variety of vegetables to dishes like stir-fries, omelets, and salads.
   - This not only boosts nutrients but also adds flavor and texture.

12. **Consultation with Healthcare Providers:**
   - Consult with healthcare providers, including registered dietitians, to determine individual dietary needs and incorporate fruits and vegetables appropriately.

13. **Educational Resources:**
   - Utilize educational resources provided by healthcare professionals to enhance your understanding of gestational diabetes management, including the role of fruits and vegetables.

14. **Individualized Approach:**
   - Customize your choices of fruits and vegetables based on personal preferences, cultural considerations, and any dietary restrictions.
   - An individualized approach enhances adherence to a healthy eating plan.

15. **Meal Planning and Preparation:**
   - Plan and prepare meals in advance, incorporating a variety of fruits and vegetables to create flavorful and well-balanced dishes.

By prioritizing a colorful array of fruits and vegetables, individuals with gestational diabetes can enjoy a wide range of nutrients while managing blood sugar levels effectively. A balanced approach, portion control, and collaboration with healthcare professionals contribute to a healthy and successful pregnancy.

CHAPTER FOUR

SNACK IDEAS

Snacking is an important aspect of managing gestational diabetes, providing a way to maintain blood sugar levels between meals. Here's a detailed explanation of snack ideas focusing on real food for gestational diabetes:

1. **Nutrient-Dense Choices:**
   - Opt for snacks that are nutrient-dense, providing essential vitamins, minerals, and fiber.
   - Nutrient-dense snacks contribute to overall health and can help stabilize blood sugar levels.

2. **Protein-Rich Snacks:**
   - Choose protein-rich snacks to support blood sugar management. Examples include:
      - Greek yogurt with berries
      - Cottage cheese with sliced cucumber
      - Hard-boiled eggs

3. **Vegetable Sticks with Hummus:**
   - Enjoy a satisfying snack by dipping vegetable sticks (carrots, celery, bell peppers) in hummus.
   - Hummus provides healthy fats and protein, while vegetables offer fiber.

4. **Nuts and Seeds:**

- Snack on a small portion of nuts (almonds, walnuts) or seeds (chia seeds, pumpkin seeds).
   - These options provide healthy fats, protein, and fiber, promoting a sense of fullness.

5. **Cheese and Whole Grain Crackers:**
   - Pairing cheese with whole grain crackers offers a combination of protein, healthy fats, and complex carbohydrates.
   - This snack provides a balance that can help stabilize blood sugar levels.

6. **Apple Slices with Nut Butter:**
   - For a filling and nutrient-dense snack, spread almond or peanut butter on apple slices.
   - The combination of fiber, healthy fats, and protein supports blood sugar control.

7. **Yogurt Parfait:**
   - Layer Greek yogurt with berries and a sprinkle of nuts or seeds for a tasty and balanced snack.
   - Greek yogurt adds protein, while berries contribute natural sweetness and fiber.

8. **Cucumber and Avocado Salad:**
   - Create a refreshing salad with cucumber slices and diced avocado.
   - Avocado provides healthy fats, and the overall snack is low in carbohydrates.

9. **Cherry Tomatoes with Mozzarella:**

- Enjoy cherry tomatoes paired with small mozzarella balls for a simple and flavorful snack.
   - This combination offers a mix of vitamins, minerals, and protein.

10. **Smoothie with Greens:**
   - Blend a smoothie with spinach or kale, berries, Greek yogurt, and a splash of almond milk.
   - Green leafy vegetables add nutrients, and the protein helps manage blood sugar levels.

11. **Edamame:**
   - Snack on steamed edamame sprinkled with a pinch of sea salt.
   - Edamame is a good source of plant-based protein and fiber.

12. **Whole Grain Toast with Avocado:**
   - Top a piece of whole grain toast with mashed avocado for a satisfying and nutritious snack.
   - The combination of healthy fats and complex carbohydrates promotes satiety.

13. **Cottage Cheese with Pineapple:**
   - Enjoy a small bowl of cottage cheese with fresh pineapple chunks.
   - Protein is provided by cottage cheese, while natural sweetness is added by pineapple.

14. **Berries with Whipped Cream:**

- Indulge in a sweet treat by combining fresh berries with a dollop of unsweetened whipped cream.
   - This dessert-like snack is relatively low in added sugars.

15. **Rice Cake with Hummus and Cherry Tomatoes:**
   - Top a rice cake with hummus and cherry tomatoes for a crunchy and satisfying snack.
   - The mix of carbohydrates, protein, and healthy fats helps maintain blood sugar levels.

16. **Cinnamon-Roasted Almonds:**
   - Roast almonds with a sprinkle of cinnamon for a flavorful and crunchy snack.
   - Cinnamon may have potential benefits for blood sugar regulation.

17. **Homemade Trail Mix:**
   - Create a personalized trail mix with a mix of nuts, seeds, and a small amount of dried fruits.
   - Portion control is key to managing overall carbohydrate intake.

18. **Hard Cheese with Whole Grain Pretzels:**
   - Pair hard cheese with whole grain pretzels for a satisfying and balanced snack.
   - The combination of protein and complex carbohydrates supports blood sugar stability.

19. **Cauliflower and Guacamole:**

- Dip cauliflower florets in guacamole for a nutritious and crunchy snack.
   - Guacamole provides healthy fats, and cauliflower is a low-carbohydrate option.

20. **Baked Sweet Potato Fries:**
   - Make baked sweet potato fries for a tasty snack that offers complex carbohydrates.
   - Pair with a protein source for added satiety.

When selecting snacks for gestational diabetes, it's crucial to focus on whole, real foods, control portion sizes, and consider the balance of macronutrients. Additionally, consulting with healthcare providers or a registered dietitian for personalized advice can help create a snack plan that aligns with individual needs and promotes optimal blood sugar management during pregnancy.

SMART SNACKING STRATEGIES

Smart snacking is crucial for individuals managing gestational diabetes, helping to stabilize blood sugar levels between meals. Here's a detailed explanation of smart snacking strategies:

1. **Balanced Macronutrients:**
   - Include a combination of carbohydrates, proteins, and healthy fats in your snacks.

- Balancing macronutrients helps manage blood sugar levels by providing a gradual release of glucose.

2. **Portion Control:**
   - Pay attention to portion sizes to avoid overconsumption of calories and carbohydrates.
   - Opt for smaller, well-portioned snacks to support blood sugar stability.

3. **Frequent, Regular Snacking:**
   - Aim for regular snacking throughout the day, spaced between main meals.
   - Frequent, smaller snacks can help prevent extreme fluctuations in blood sugar levels.

4. **Timing Matters:**
   - Schedule snacks strategically between meals to maintain a steady energy supply.
   - Consistent timing can contribute to better blood sugar control.

5. **Whole, Real Foods:**
   - Choose whole, minimally processed foods for snacks to maximize nutrient intake.
   - Whole foods, such as fruits, vegetables, nuts, and lean proteins, provide essential nutrients and support overall health.

6. **Fiber-Rich Choices:**
   - Select snacks high in fiber, such as fruits, vegetables, and whole grains.

   - Fiber helps to maintain stable blood sugar levels by slowing down the absorption of glucose.

7. **Hydration:**
   - Stay well-hydrated by sipping water between snacks.
   - Sipping enough water promotes general health and helps you feel fuller.

8. **Preparation and Planning:**
   - Plan your snacks in advance to ensure you have nutritious options readily available.
   - Preparation helps avoid reaching for less healthy, convenient choices.

9. **Mindful Eating:**
   - Eat mindfully by appreciating every taste and being aware of your body's signals of hunger and fullness.
   - Being mindful can help prevent overeating and promote satisfaction.

10. **Low-Glycemic Options:**
   - Choose snacks with a low glycemic index to minimize their impact on blood sugar levels.
   - Low-GI options include most non-starchy vegetables, berries, and certain whole grains.

11. **Avoiding Added Sugars:**
   - Minimize or avoid snacks with added sugars to prevent unnecessary spikes in blood sugar.

- To find hidden sugars in packaged foods, read the labels.

12. **Protein-Packed Choices:**
   - Prioritize protein-rich snacks to promote satiety and stabilize blood sugar levels.
   - Lean meats, nuts, seeds, cottage cheese, and Greek yogurt are among the options.

13. **Monitoring Blood Sugar Levels:**
   - Regularly monitor your blood sugar levels to understand how different snacks affect your body.
   - Use this information to make informed choices and adjust your snack plan as needed.

14. **Physical Activity:**
   - Incorporate light physical activity after snacks, such as a short walk.
   - Physical activity can assist in glucose regulation and overall well-being.

15. **Individualized Approach:**
   - Customize your snacking approach based on your preferences, dietary needs, and lifestyle.
   - An individualized strategy enhances adherence to a healthy eating plan.

16. **Educational Resources:**
   - Utilize educational resources provided by healthcare professionals to enhance your understanding of gestational diabetes management, including smart snacking.

17. **Consultation with Healthcare Providers:**
   - Consult with healthcare providers, including registered dietitians, to receive personalized guidance on smart snacking strategies.
   - Healthcare professionals can tailor advice to your specific needs and monitor your overall health during pregnancy.

By incorporating these smart snacking strategies, individuals with gestational diabetes can maintain stable blood sugar levels, support overall health, and ensure a successful and healthy pregnancy.

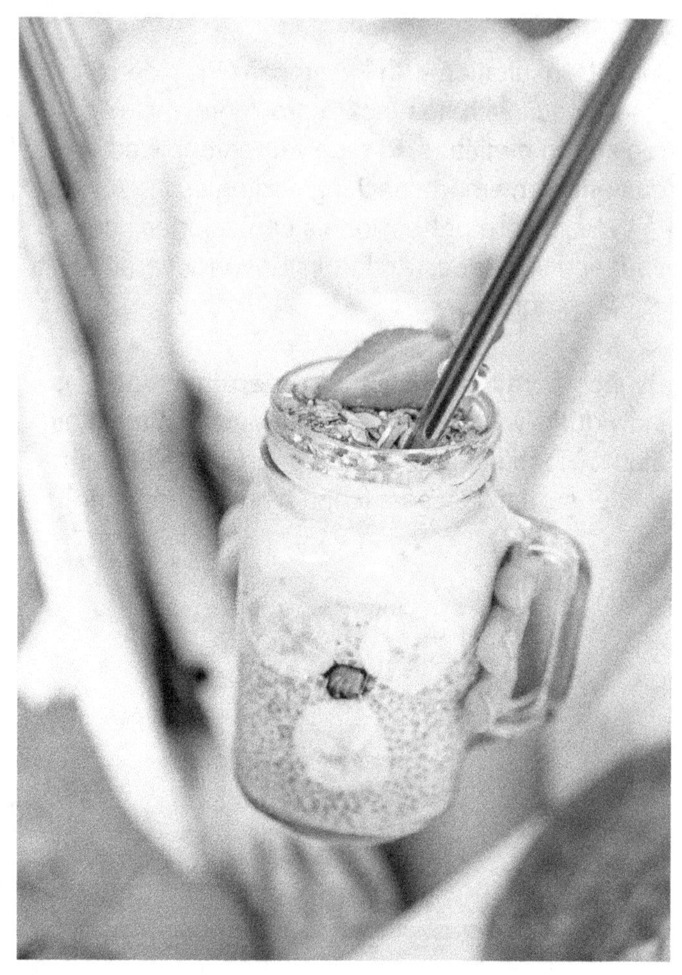

CHAPTER FIVE

RECIPE COLLECTION

Creating a collection of recipes tailored for gestational diabetes involves selecting nutrient-dense ingredients that support blood sugar control while providing essential nutrients for both the mother and baby. Here's a detailed explanation on building a recipe collection for gestational diabetes:

1. **Focus on Whole, Real Foods:**
   - Emphasize recipes that feature whole, minimally processed foods such as fruits, vegetables, lean proteins, whole grains, and healthy fats.
   - Whole foods provide essential nutrients and fiber, promoting overall health.

2. **Balanced Macronutrients:**
   - Design recipes that include a balance of carbohydrates, proteins, and healthy fats.
   - Balancing macronutrients helps manage blood sugar levels and provides sustained energy.

3. **Portion Control:**
   - Ensure recipes include appropriate portion sizes to help control overall calorie and carbohydrate intake.
   - Controlling portion sizes is essential for keeping blood sugar levels steady.

4. **Low-Glycemic Options:**
   - Incorporate ingredients with a low glycemic index to minimize their impact on blood sugar levels.
   - Low-GI options include most non-starchy vegetables, legumes, and certain whole grains.

5. **Fiber-Rich Ingredients:**
   - Choose ingredients high in fiber, such as whole grains, vegetables, and legumes.
   - Fiber aids digestion and slows down the absorption of glucose, supporting blood sugar stability.

6. **Lean Proteins:**
   - Include lean protein sources in recipes, such as poultry, fish, tofu, legumes, and lean cuts of meat.
   - Protein helps maintain satiety and supports fetal development.

7. **Healthy Fats:**
   - Integrate sources of healthy fats, like avocados, nuts, seeds, and olive oil, into recipes.
   - Healthy fats are essential for fetal brain development and overall maternal health.

8. **Mindful Cooking Methods:**
   - Opt for cooking methods that preserve the nutritional value of ingredients, such as baking, grilling, steaming, or sautéing.
   - Minimize frying or cooking with excessive oils.

9. **Flavorful Herbs and Spices:**
   - Use herbs and spices to add flavor without relying on excessive salt, sugar, or unhealthy condiments.
   - Experimenting with various herbs and spices enhances the sensory appeal of dishes.

10. **Meal Diversity:**
   - Create a diverse collection of recipes to prevent dietary monotony.
   - Explore different cuisines, cooking styles, and flavor profiles to keep meals interesting.

11. **Hydration Incorporation:**
   - Integrate hydrating ingredients into recipes, such as soups, stews, and fruit-infused water.
   - Maintaining adequate hydration promotes general health and facilitates digestion.

12. **Batch Cooking and Freezing:**
   - Consider recipes that can be prepared in batches and frozen for convenient, time-saving meal options.
   - Batch cooking ensures you have nutritious meals readily available.

13. **Nutritional Information:**
   - Include nutritional information for each recipe, such as total carbohydrates, proteins, fats, and fiber.

- This information assists in meal planning and adherence to dietary recommendations.

14. **Collaboration with Healthcare Professionals:**
   - Collaborate with healthcare providers, including registered dietitians, to ensure the recipes align with individual dietary needs and health goals.
   - Healthcare professionals can provide personalized guidance based on specific health considerations.

15. **Educational Resources:**
   - Utilize educational resources provided by healthcare professionals or reputable sources to enhance your understanding of gestational diabetes management through nutrition.
   - Educational materials can offer insights into the nutritional requirements during pregnancy.

16. **Community Support:**
   - Connect with support groups or communities focused on gestational diabetes for recipe sharing and inspiration.
   - Sharing experiences and recipe ideas with others can provide valuable insights and encouragement.

17. **Ingredient Substitutions:**
   - Identify and incorporate healthy ingredient substitutions to accommodate individual preferences and dietary restrictions.

- Substituting ingredients can enhance the nutritional profile of recipes.

18. **Variety in Texture and Flavors:**
   - Aim for recipes with a variety of textures and flavors to make meals more enjoyable.
   - Exploring different culinary elements adds excitement to the dining experience.

19. **Feedback and Adaptation:**
   - Collect feedback from personal experiences and adapt recipes based on taste preferences, nutritional needs, and overall satisfaction.
   - Regularly revisiting and refining your recipe collection ensures it remains dynamic and well-suited to your needs.

20. **Meal Planning Integration:**
   - Integrate the recipes into a comprehensive meal planning strategy to ensure a well-balanced and varied diet.
   - Meal planning enhances organization and supports consistent adherence to dietary guidelines.

Building a recipe collection for gestational diabetes involves a thoughtful selection of ingredients, cooking methods, and nutritional considerations. By prioritizing nutrient-dense, whole foods and collaborating with healthcare professionals, individuals can create a versatile and enjoyable

collection of recipes that align with the specific
needs of gestational diabetes management.

BREAKFAST

Certainly! Here's a simple and nutritious breakfast
idea suitable for gestational diabetes:

**Vegetable and Cheese Omelet with Whole Grain
Toast:**

Ingredients:
- 2 large eggs
- 1/4 cup diced bell peppers (any color)
- 1/4 cup diced tomatoes
- 1/4 cup diced onions
- 1/4 cup shredded low-fat cheese (cheddar or
mozzarella)
- 1 teaspoon olive oil
- Salt and pepper to taste
- 1 slice of whole grain bread

Instructions:
1. In a bowl, whisk the eggs and season with a
pinch of salt and pepper.
2. In a nonstick skillet, preheat the olive oil over
medium heat.
3. Add diced bell peppers, tomatoes, and onions to
the skillet. Sauté until vegetables are tender.
4. Pour the whisked eggs over the sautéed
vegetables in the skillet.

5. Allow the eggs to set slightly around the edges, then gently lift the edges with a spatula to let the uncooked eggs flow underneath.
6. Once the eggs are mostly set, sprinkle shredded cheese over one half of the omelet.
7. Fold the omelet in half, covering the cheese, and cook for an additional minute until the cheese melts and the eggs are fully cooked.
8. Toast a slice of whole grain bread.
9. Serve the omelet with the whole grain toast on the side.

This breakfast choice offers a balanced intake of healthy fats, protein, and carbohydrates. The whole grain toast adds fiber, while the vegetables contribute essential vitamins and minerals. The eggs and cheese provide protein for satiety and fetal development. Adjust portion sizes based on individual dietary needs, and as always, consult with healthcare providers for personalized advice.

LUNCH

Certainly! Here's a nutritious and balanced lunch idea suitable for gestational diabetes:

Grilled Chicken Salad with Quinoa:

Ingredients:

For the Salad:

- 4 oz grilled chicken breast, sliced
- 2 cups mixed salad greens (spinach, arugula, or
your choice)
- 1/2 cup cherry tomatoes, halved
- 1/4 cucumber, sliced
- 1/4 cup shredded carrots
- 1/4 cup feta cheese, crumbled (optional)
- 2 tablespoons sliced almonds

For the Quinoa:
- 1/2 cup quinoa, rinsed
- 1 cup water
- Pinch of salt

For the Dressing:
- 2 tablespoons olive oil
- 1 tablespoon balsamic vinegar
- 1 teaspoon Dijon mustard
- Salt and pepper to taste

Instructions:

1. **Prepare the Quinoa:**
   - In a saucepan, combine quinoa, water, and a
pinch of salt.
   - Once the quinoa is cooked and the water has
been absorbed, reduce the heat to low, cover, and
simmer for 15 minutes.
   - Using a fork, fluff the quinoa and set aside to
chill.

2. **Grill the Chicken:**

- Season the chicken breast with salt and pepper.
- Grill the chicken until fully cooked, approximately 5-7 minutes per side, depending on thickness.
- Slice the grilled chicken into strips.

3. **Assemble the Salad:**
   - In a large bowl, combine the mixed salad greens, cherry tomatoes, cucumber, shredded carrots, and sliced almonds.
   - Add the sliced grilled chicken on top.
   - Add some crumbled feta cheese to the salad if you'd like.

4. **Make the Dressing:**
   - In a small bowl, whisk together olive oil, balsamic vinegar, Dijon mustard, salt, and pepper.

5. **Assemble the Lunch:**
   - Arrange a portion of the salad onto a dish.
   - Add a portion of the cooked quinoa on the side.
   - Drizzle the dressing over the salad and quinoa.

This lunch option offers a mix of lean protein, fiber-rich vegetables, and whole grains. The quinoa provides complex carbohydrates, and the grilled chicken contributes essential proteins. The salad greens, vegetables, and almonds add vitamins, minerals, and healthy fats. Adjust portion sizes based on individual dietary needs, and consult with healthcare providers for personalized advice.

Certainly! Here's a wholesome and balanced dinner idea suitable for gestational diabetes:

Grilled Salmon with Quinoa and Roasted Vegetables:

Ingredients:

For the Grilled Salmon:
- 1 lb salmon fillets
- 1 tablespoon olive oil
- Lemon juice
- Dill (fresh or dried)
- Salt and pepper to taste

For the Quinoa:
- 1 cup quinoa, rinsed
- 2 cups water
- Pinch of salt

For the Roasted Vegetables:
- 2 cups mixed vegetables (bell peppers, cherry tomatoes, zucchini, broccoli)
- 1 tablespoon olive oil
- Garlic powder
- Italian seasoning
- Salt and pepper to taste

Instructions:

1. **Preheat the Oven:**
   - Set oven temperature to 200°C, or 400°F.

2. **Prepare the Quinoa:**
   - In a saucepan, combine quinoa, water, and a pinch of salt.
   - Bring to a boil, then reduce heat to low, cover, and simmer for 15 minutes or until quinoa is cooked and water is absorbed.
   - Set aside the quinoa after fluffing it with a fork.

3. **Prepare the Roasted Vegetables:**
   - Toss mixed vegetables with olive oil, garlic powder, Italian seasoning, salt, and pepper.
   - Arrange the veggies evenly onto a baking sheet.
   - Roast in the preheated oven for 20-25 minutes or until vegetables are tender and slightly browned.

4. **Grill the Salmon:**
   - Brush salmon fillets with olive oil and lemon juice.
   - Sprinkle dill, salt, and pepper over the salmon.
   - The salmon should flake easily with a fork after grilling it for about 4–5 minutes on each side.

5. **Assemble the Dinner:**
   - Place a portion of quinoa on each plate.
   - Top with grilled salmon fillets.
   - Serve with a generous portion of roasted vegetables on the side.

Additional Tips:

- Garnish the salmon with fresh lemon slices for added flavor.
- Consider adding a drizzle of olive oil or a squeeze of lemon juice to the quinoa for extra zest.
- Adjust seasoning to taste preferences.

This dinner option provides a balance of lean protein from the salmon, complex carbohydrates from quinoa, and a variety of vitamins and minerals from the colorful roasted vegetables. Always adjust portion sizes based on individual dietary needs, and consult with healthcare providers for personalized advice on gestational diabetes management.

SNACKS AND DESSERTS

Certainly! Here are snack and dessert ideas suitable for gestational diabetes:

Snack Idea: Greek Yogurt Parfait

Ingredients:
- 1/2 cup plain Greek yogurt
- berries (blueberries, strawberries, or raspberries) 1/4 cup
- 1 tablespoon chia seeds
- 1 tablespoon of finely chopped nuts (walnuts or almonds)
- 1 teaspoon honey (optional for sweetness)

Instructions:

1. In a bowl or glass, layer Greek yogurt with berries.
2. Sprinkle chia seeds and chopped nuts over the yogurt.
3. Drizzle with honey if desired.
4. Mix before eating to combine flavors and textures.

Snack Idea: Hummus and Veggie Sticks

Ingredients:
- 1/4 cup hummus
- Carrot sticks, cucumber slices, and bell pepper strips for dipping

Instructions:
1. Arrange the veggie sticks on a plate.
2. Serve with hummus for a satisfying and nutrient-dense snack.

Snack Idea: Apple Slices with Peanut Butter

Ingredients:
- 1 medium apple, sliced
- 2 tablespoons natural peanut butter

Instructions:
1. Spread peanut butter on apple slices.
2. Enjoy the combination of sweetness and protein.

Dessert Idea: Berry and Greek Yogurt Popsicles

Ingredients:
- One cup of mixed berries, including raspberries, blueberries, and strawberries
- 1 cup plain Greek yogurt
- 1-2 tablespoons honey (optional for sweetness)

Instructions:
1. In a blender, puree the berries until smooth.
2. In a separate bowl, mix Greek yogurt with honey.
3. Layer the berry puree and yogurt mixture in popsicle molds.
4. Put the popsicle sticks in and freeze until they solidify.

Dessert Idea: Dark Chocolate and Almond Clusters

Ingredients:
- 1/2 cup dark chocolate chips (70% cocoa or higher)
- 1/2 cup almonds, whole or chopped

Instructions:
1. In a heatproof basin, melt the dark chocolate.
2. Stir in almonds until well coated.
3. Drop spoonfuls onto a parchment-lined tray.
4. Allow to cool until chocolate hardens.

Remember to monitor portion sizes, choose snacks and desserts with balanced macronutrients, and consider individual dietary preferences. As always, consult with healthcare providers or a registered dietitian for personalized guidance based on specific health needs and gestational diabetes management.

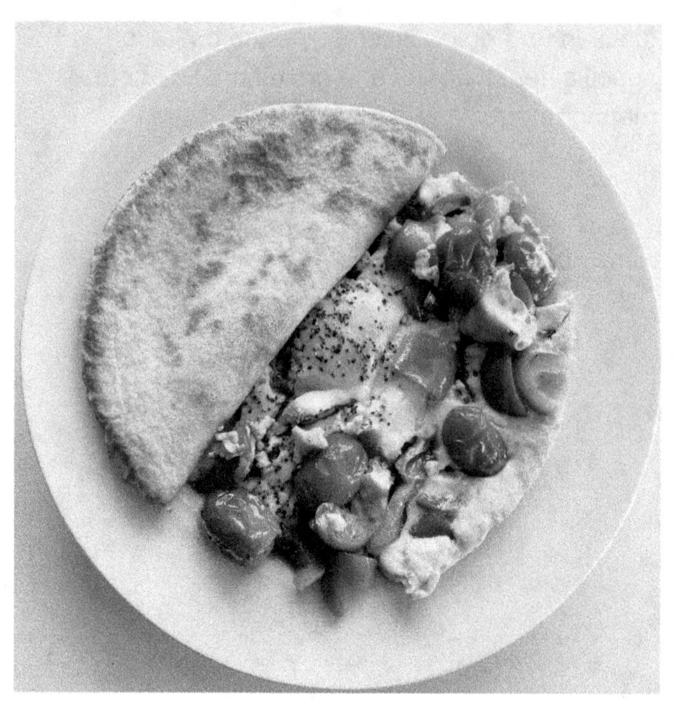

CHAPTER SIX

EATING OUT TIPS

Eating out while managing gestational diabetes can be manageable with some thoughtful choices. Here are some tips for making healthier choices when dining out:

1. **Plan Ahead:**
   - Check the restaurant's menu online in advance, if possible, to identify healthier options.

2. **Choose Grilled or Baked Proteins:**
   - Opt for grilled, baked, or broiled lean proteins like chicken, fish, or lean cuts of beef.

3. **Watch Portion Sizes:**
   - Pay attention to portion sizes, and consider sharing a dish or taking leftovers home.

4. **Select Whole Grains:**
   - Choose whole grains when possible, such as brown rice, quinoa, or whole grain pasta.

5. **Load Up on Vegetables:**
   - Include a variety of vegetables in your meal for added fiber and nutrients.

6. **Limit Added Sugars:**

- Be cautious of dishes with added sugars. To regulate the quantity, ask for dressings and sauces on the side.

7. **Choose Water or Unsweetened Beverages:**
   - Opt for water, herbal tea, or other unsweetened beverages instead of sugary drinks.

8. **Ask for Modifications:**
   - Don't hesitate to ask for modifications, such as steaming or grilling instead of frying.

9. **Skip Fried and Breaded Options:**
   - Avoid fried and breaded dishes, as they can be higher in unhealthy fats and carbohydrates.

10. **Be Mindful of Sauces and Condiments:**
    - Choose sauces and condiments sparingly, as they can contribute to added calories and sugars.

11. **Monitor Alcohol Intake:**
    - If you choose to have alcohol, do so in moderation and consider lower-sugar options.

12. **Control Your Carb Intake:**
    - Be mindful of your carbohydrate intake, and balance it with protein and vegetables.

13. **Consider Salads with Protein:**
    - Opt for salads with lean protein sources and choose vinaigrette dressings on the side.

14. **Ask Questions:**
   - Don't hesitate to ask the waiter about how dishes are prepared and if modifications are possible.

15. **Practice Portion Control:**
   - Use visual cues or ask for a smaller portion if the regular serving size is too large.

16. **Stay Hydrated:**
   - Drink water throughout the meal to help with hydration and control appetite.

17. **Skip the Bread Basket:**
   - Consider skipping the bread basket to reduce overall carbohydrate intake.

18. **Choose Fresh Fruit for Dessert:**
   - If you decide to have dessert, opt for fresh fruit or a small portion of a lower-sugar option.

Remember to monitor your blood sugar levels regularly, especially if you're trying new foods or making adjustments to your routine. Always consult with your healthcare team or a registered dietitian for personalized advice based on your individual needs and gestational diabetes management.

MAKING HEALTHY CHOICES

Making healthy choices is essential for managing gestational diabetes and promoting overall well-being. The following are some broad pointers for selecting nutritious foods:

1. **Choose Whole, Unprocessed Foods:**
   - Give entire foods like fruits, vegetables, whole grains, lean meats, and healthy fats priority.

2. **Opt for Balanced Meals:**
   - Include a mix of carbohydrates, proteins, and fats in each meal to help stabilize blood sugar levels.

3. **Control Portion Sizes:**
   - Be mindful of portion sizes to manage calorie and carbohydrate intake. Reduce the size of your plates to aid in portion control.

4. **Prioritize Fiber-Rich Foods:**
   - Include high-fiber foods like vegetables, fruits, whole grains, and legumes to promote satiety and stabilize blood sugar.

5. **Limit Added Sugars and Refined Carbs:**
   - Avoid sugary beverages, candies, and heavily processed foods. Choose whole grains over refined grains.

6. **Include Lean Proteins:**

- Incorporate lean protein sources such as poultry, fish, tofu, legumes, and low-fat dairy to support muscle health.

7. **Choose Healthy Fats:**
   - Incorporate, but in moderation, foods high in unsaturated fats, such as avocados, nuts, seeds, and olive oil.

8. **Stay Hydrated:**
   - Drink plenty of water throughout the day, herbal tea, or infused water instead of sugar-filled beverages.

9. **Spread Meals and Snacks:**
   - Eat regular, balanced meals and snacks throughout the day to help manage blood sugar levels.

10. **Be Mindful of Cooking Methods:**
    - Instead of frying, use healthier cooking techniques like grilling, baking, steaming, or sautéing.

11. **Read Food Labels:**
    - Check food labels for nutritional information, paying attention to total carbohydrates, fiber, and added sugars.

12. **Plan Ahead:**
    - Plan meals and snacks in advance to ensure balanced and nutritious choices.

13. **Monitor Blood Sugar Levels:**
   - Regularly check your blood sugar levels as recommended by your healthcare team to track how food choices affect your body.

14. **Incorporate Physical Activity:**
   - Get regular exercise; this can help with blood sugar regulation and insulin sensitivity.

15. **Get Support:**
   - Seek guidance and support from healthcare providers, including dietitians or nutritionists, to create a personalized and sustainable eating plan.

16. **Practice Mindful Eating:**
   - Be mindful of signals of hunger and fullness. Avoid distractions while eating to savor and enjoy your meals.

17. **Include Variety:**
   - To guarantee a wide variety of nutrients, aim for a varied assortment of foods.

18. **Manage Stress:**
   - Practice stress-reducing techniques, as stress can impact blood sugar levels.

Remember, individual needs may vary, so it's crucial to work closely with your healthcare team to create a plan that aligns with your specific health condition and lifestyle. Making small, gradual changes can lead to long-term success in maintaining a healthy and balanced diet during gestational diabetes.

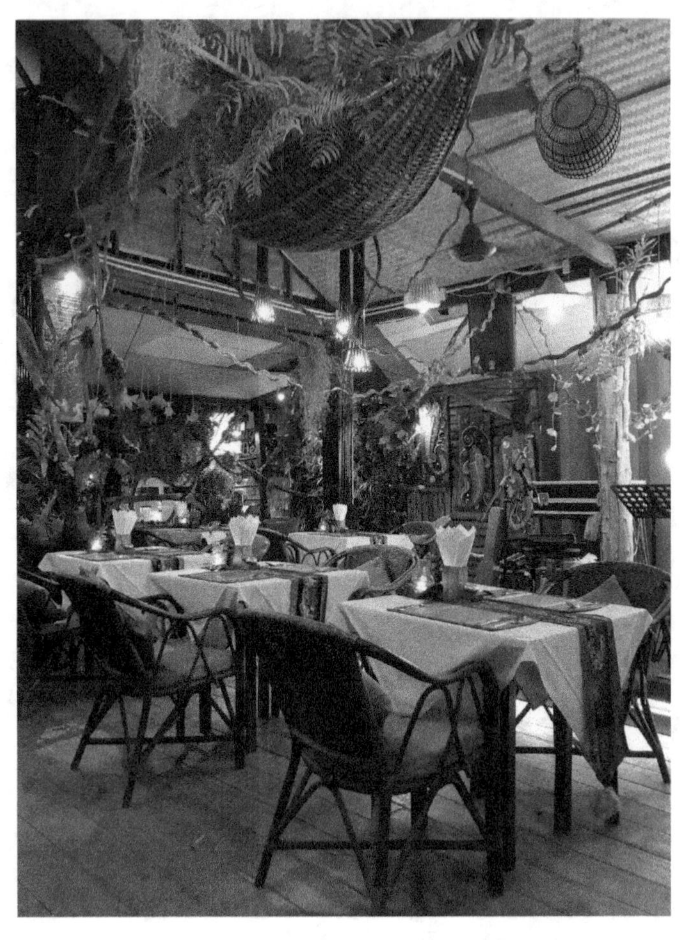

CHAPTER SEVEN

PHYSICAL ACTIVITY

Physical activity during pregnancy is a vital component of maintaining overall health and well-being for both the expectant mother and the developing fetus. Engaging in regular exercise can offer a range of benefits, including improved cardiovascular health, enhanced mood, better sleep, and potential relief from common discomforts associated with pregnancy. However, it's crucial to approach physical activity during this time with care and consideration.

Benefits of Physical Activity during Pregnancy:

1. **Cardiovascular Health:**
   - Regular exercise helps improve cardiovascular function, reducing the risk of gestational hypertension and preeclampsia.

2. **Mood Regulation:**
   - Physical activity releases endorphins, contributing to improved mood and reduced stress levels.

3. **Gestational Diabetes Management:**
   - Exercise can aid in managing gestational diabetes by improving insulin sensitivity and glucose metabolism.

4. **Weight Management:**
   - Maintaining a healthy weight through exercise supports overall health and reduces the risk of complications.

5. **Muscle Strength and Endurance:**
   - Strengthening exercises, particularly focusing on the core and pelvic floor muscles, can help alleviate back pain and improve posture.

6. **Preparation for Labor:**
   - Endurance exercises, such as walking and swimming, contribute to increased stamina, potentially aiding in the labor and delivery process.

7. **Improved Sleep:**
   - Regular physical activity is associated with better sleep quality, a common concern for pregnant individuals.

Considerations for Safe Physical Activity:

1. **Consultation with Healthcare Providers:**
   - Before initiating or continuing an exercise routine, it is crucial to consult with healthcare providers to ensure the safety of both the mother and the baby.

2. **Appropriate Exercise Selection:**

- Opt for low-impact activities, such as walking, swimming, stationary cycling, and prenatal yoga, to minimize stress on joints.

3. **Monitoring Intensity:**
   - Maintain moderate-intensity exercise, gauging effort through perceived exertion rather than heart rate. Avoid activities that lead to exhaustion.

4. **Hydration:**
   - Stay well-hydrated before, during, and after exercise to prevent dehydration and maintain body temperature.

5. **Body Awareness:**
   - Listen to the body's cues and modify or stop activities if discomfort, pain, dizziness, or shortness of breath occurs.

6. **Prenatal Classes:**
   - Consider participating in prenatal exercise classes or programs designed by fitness professionals with expertise in pregnancy fitness.

7. **Pelvic Floor Exercises:**
   - Incorporate pelvic floor exercises (Kegels) to support pelvic health and potentially reduce the risk of urinary incontinence.

8. **Adaptations as Pregnancy Progresses:**
   - Modify exercises as the pregnancy progresses, avoiding lying flat on the back after the first

trimester and being cautious with activities that involve balance.

Final Thoughts:

Engaging in regular physical activity during pregnancy is not only safe but often highly encouraged for its numerous health benefits. However, each pregnancy is unique, and individual considerations, medical history, and any potential complications must be taken into account. The key is to approach physical activity with mindfulness, seeking guidance from healthcare providers to create a personalized exercise plan that aligns with the individual's health status and pregnancy condition.

SAFE EXERCISE OPTIONS

Choosing safe exercise options during pregnancy is crucial to promote maternal health and well-being without posing risks to the developing fetus. Here are some safe exercise options for pregnant individuals, considering the various stages of pregnancy:

1. **Walking:**
   - An excellent low-impact exercise that is gentle on the joints and can be easily adapted to different fitness levels. It promotes cardiovascular health and can be continued throughout pregnancy.

2. **Swimming:**
   - Swimming and water aerobics provide a full-body workout with minimal impact on joints. The buoyancy of the water reduces strain and supports the growing belly.

3. **Prenatal Yoga:**
   - Specifically designed for pregnant women, prenatal yoga focuses on gentle stretching, relaxation, and breathing exercises. It helps improve flexibility and promotes relaxation.

4. **Prenatal Pilates:**
   - Similar to yoga, prenatal Pilates emphasizes core strength, flexibility, and overall muscle tone. It can be adapted to various fitness levels and stages of pregnancy.

5. **Stationary Cycling:**
   - Riding a stationary bike is a low-impact way to get cardiovascular exercise. Adjust the resistance to a comfortable level and maintain an upright posture.

6. **Low-Impact Aerobics:**
   - Participating in low-impact aerobics classes designed for pregnant women can be a safe way to improve cardiovascular fitness and muscle tone.

7. **Strength Training with Modifications:**

   - Incorporate light to moderate strength training with a focus on proper form. Use lighter weights and perform more repetitions. After the first trimester, avoid resting flat on your back.

8. **Prenatal Fitness Classes:**
   - Attend prenatal fitness classes led by certified instructors who specialize in pregnancy exercise. These classes often combine a variety of safe and effective exercises.

9. **Kegel Exercises:**
   - Strengthening the pelvic floor muscles through Kegel exercises can help prevent urinary incontinence and support pelvic health. These exercises can be done at any time of day.

10. **Gentle Stretching:**
   - Include gentle stretching exercises to improve flexibility and alleviate tension. Focus on major muscle groups while avoiding overstretching.

11. **Breathing Exercises:**
   - Incorporate deep breathing exercises to promote relaxation and reduce stress. Breathing techniques can also be beneficial during labor.

12. **Dancing:**
   - Participate in low-impact dance classes or dance to your favorite music at home. Ensure movements are controlled, and avoid high-impact jumps or sudden twists.

13. **Modified Planks:**
   - If accustomed to planks, consider modified plank positions that engage the core without putting excess strain on the abdomen. Always prioritize proper form.

14. **Tai Chi:**
   - Tai Chi is a low-impact, gentle form of exercise that promotes balance, flexibility, and relaxation. It can be adapted for pregnancy.

15. **Elliptical Trainer:**
   - An elliptical machine can be used to work out your cardiovascular system with minimal impact. Adjust the resistance to a comfortable level and maintain proper posture.

Remember to listen to your body, stay hydrated, and avoid activities that cause discomfort, pain, dizziness, or shortness of breath. Always consult with your healthcare provider before starting any exercise program during pregnancy, especially if you have specific health concerns or complications.

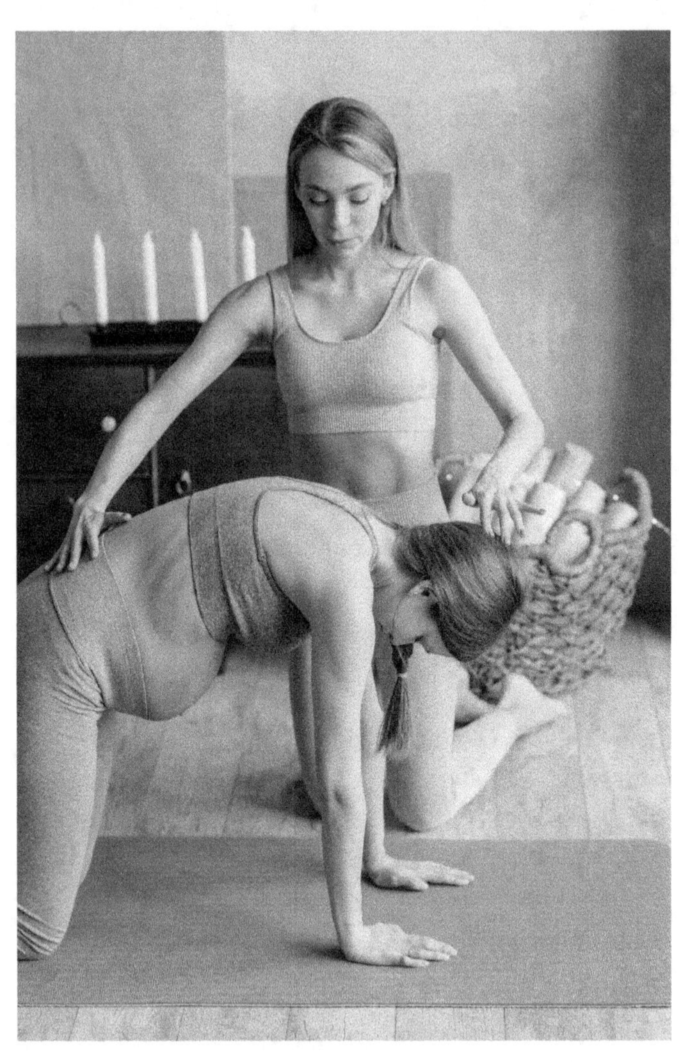

CHAPTER EIGHT

MONITORING BLOOD SUGAR

Blood sugar monitoring is an essential part of controlling gestational diabetes. Regular monitoring helps individuals understand how their lifestyle, including dietary choices and physical activity, impacts blood glucose levels. Here's a guide on monitoring blood sugar during pregnancy:

1. **Frequency of Monitoring:**
   - Adhere to your healthcare provider's monitoring routine. This typically involves checking blood sugar levels multiple times a day, such as before and after meals.

2. **Testing Times:**
   - Common testing times include fasting (before breakfast) and postprandial (after meals). Your healthcare professional will provide you precise instructions depending on your personal needs.

3. **Blood Glucose Targets:**
   - Be aware of your target blood glucose levels, as advised by your healthcare team. These targets may vary depending on whether you are testing fasting or postprandial levels.

4. **Using a Glucometer:**

- Invest in a reliable glucometer. Your healthcare provider or diabetes educator will guide you on its proper use. It typically involves pricking your finger to obtain a small blood sample, which is then analyzed by the glucometer.

5. **Recording Results:**
   - Keep a record of your blood sugar levels. Note the time of day, the value of the reading, and any relevant details such as the type of meal you consumed or recent physical activity.

6. **Pattern Recognition:**
   - Review your blood sugar log regularly to identify patterns. This can help you and your healthcare team make informed adjustments to your diet, exercise routine, or medication if needed.

7. **Understanding Glycemic Index:**
   - Be aware of the glycemic index of foods. Foods with a lower glycemic index release glucose more slowly, helping to avoid rapid spikes in blood sugar.

8. **Meal Timing:**
   - Spread out your meals and snacks throughout the day. Consistent meal timing can contribute to better blood sugar control.

9. **Carbohydrate Monitoring:**
   - Pay attention to carbohydrate intake, as it has a direct impact on blood sugar levels. Your healthcare

team can guide you on appropriate carbohydrate portions.

10. **Postprandial Monitoring:**
   - Monitoring blood sugar after meals is essential. This helps identify how different foods affect your body and allows for adjustments in meal planning.

11. **Hydration:**
   - Stay hydrated. Dehydration can affect blood sugar levels, so ensure you are drinking enough water throughout the day.

12. **Consultation with Healthcare Providers:**
   - Share your blood sugar log with your healthcare team during regular appointments. This information helps them provide personalized guidance based on your specific needs and responses to treatment.

13. **Medication Adherence:**
   - If you are given medication, take it exactly as advised by your doctor. Regular blood sugar monitoring helps ensure that medication is effectively managing glucose levels.

14. **Emergency Situations:**
   - Know what to do in case of extremely high or low blood sugar levels. Follow the guidance provided by your healthcare team for managing these situations.

Remember, gestational diabetes management is highly individualized, and your healthcare provider will tailor recommendations to your specific situation. Regular communication with your healthcare team is essential for effective blood sugar control and a healthy pregnancy.

TIPS FOR REGULAR MONITORING

Certainly! Here are some practical tips for regular monitoring of blood sugar levels during gestational diabetes:

1. **Set a Schedule:**
   - Establish a consistent schedule for monitoring, including specific times for fasting (before breakfast) and postprandial (after meals) readings.

2. **Use Reminders:**
   - Set alarms or reminders on your phone to prompt you to check blood sugar at designated times. Consistency is key in managing gestational diabetes.

3. **Keep Supplies Handy:**
   - Ensure you have your glucometer, test strips, lancets, and a logbook or app readily available. Having everything in one place makes it easier to stick to your monitoring routine.

4. **Create a Comfortable Space:**

- Choose a comfortable and well-lit area for testing. Being in a calm environment can help reduce stress, which may affect blood sugar levels.

5. **Rotate Testing Sites:**
   - Rotate the finger you use for blood sampling to avoid discomfort and minimize the risk of developing calluses or sore spots.

6. **Practice Good Hand Hygiene:**
   - To ensure reliable readings, properly wash your hands before testing. Avoid using alcohol-based hand sanitizers right before testing, as they can affect results.

7. **Follow Proper Technique:**
   - Adhere to the recommended technique for using your glucometer. Ensure your hands and the testing area are clean, and use the appropriate lancet depth setting to obtain an adequate blood sample.

8. **Vary Test Times:**
   - Occasionally vary the times at which you check your blood sugar levels, especially postprandial readings. This provides a more comprehensive understanding of your glucose control throughout the day.

9. **Record Relevant Details:**
   - In your logbook or app, record not only blood sugar values but also details about meals, snacks,

physical activity, and any other factors that may influence glucose levels.

10. **Stay Hydrated:**
   - Maintain proper hydration, as dehydration can impact blood sugar levels. Drink water regularly, especially before and after testing.

11. **Review Patterns:**
   - Regularly review your blood sugar log to identify patterns or trends. This can help you and your healthcare team make informed decisions about adjustments to your diet or treatment plan.

12. **Seek Support:**
   - Share your monitoring routine with a family member or friend who can provide support and encouragement. Having someone to share your experiences with can be beneficial.

13. **Stay Positive:**
   - Acknowledge that blood sugar levels can fluctuate, and occasional readings outside the target range may occur. Stay positive and focus on making adjustments to improve overall control.

14. **Ask for Help:**
   - If you encounter challenges or have concerns about your monitoring routine, don't hesitate to reach out to your healthcare provider or diabetes educator for guidance.

15. **Celebrate Achievements:**
   - Celebrate successes, whether it's consistently hitting target ranges or making positive changes in response to your blood sugar monitoring.

Remember that monitoring blood sugar levels is a valuable tool for managing gestational diabetes, and with time and practice, it becomes a routine part of your pregnancy journey. If you ever have questions or encounter difficulties, don't hesitate to reach out to your healthcare team for guidance and support.

UNDERSTANDING RESULTS

Understanding blood sugar results is crucial for managing gestational diabetes effectively. Here's a breakdown of common blood sugar readings and what they may indicate:

1. **Fasting Blood Sugar (Before Breakfast):**
   - **Normal Range:** Typically, less than 95 mg/dL.
   - **Target for Gestational Diabetes:** Your healthcare provider will provide a specific target, often aiming for values below 90 mg/dL.

2. **Postprandial Blood Sugar (After Meals):**
   - **Normal Range:** Typically, less than 140 mg/dL two hours after a meal.

- **Target for Gestational Diabetes:** Your healthcare provider may recommend postprandial values below 120 mg/dL or provide personalized targets.

3. **Understanding Targets:**
  - Targets can vary, and your healthcare team will set specific goals based on your individual health, gestational age, and other factors. Always follow the targets provided by your healthcare provider.

4. **Interpreting Readings:**
  - **Within Target Range:** This indicates good blood sugar control and aligns with your treatment plan. Continue with your current management approach.
  - **Above Target Range:** Consult with your healthcare provider. They may recommend adjustments to your diet, physical activity, or medication.
  - **Consistently Low Readings:** This could indicate hypoglycemia. If you experience symptoms such as dizziness or shakiness, contact your healthcare provider.

5. **Patterns and Trends:**
  - Regularly review your blood sugar log to identify patterns. Note if certain meals consistently lead to higher or lower readings. This information helps refine your management plan.

6. **Consult with Healthcare Team:**

- Always consult with your healthcare provider if you have questions or concerns about your blood sugar readings. They can provide personalized guidance and adjustments to your treatment plan.

7. **Medication Adjustments:**
   - If you are taking medication to manage gestational diabetes, your healthcare provider may adjust the dosage based on your blood sugar readings. Never alter your medication without consulting them.

8. **Meal Timing and Composition:**
   - Note the impact of different meals on your blood sugar. This information can guide meal planning, helping you make choices that align with your targets.

9. **Physical Activity:**
   - Regular physical activity can influence blood sugar levels. Take note of how exercise affects your readings and discuss any concerns with your healthcare provider.

10. **Stress and Sleep:**
   - Emotional stress and inadequate sleep can impact blood sugar levels. Be mindful of these factors and discuss strategies for managing stress with your healthcare team.

Remember that gestational diabetes management is individualized, and your healthcare provider will tailor recommendations to your specific situation. Regular communication with your healthcare team is essential for interpreting results, making adjustments as needed, and ensuring the best possible outcomes for both you and your baby.

CONCLUSION

In conclusion, managing gestational diabetes is a dynamic process that involves a combination of regular blood sugar monitoring, thoughtful meal planning, physical activity, and collaboration with your healthcare team. The key elements for a successful management plan include:

1. **Consistent Monitoring:**
   - Regularly monitor your blood sugar levels according to the schedule recommended by your healthcare provider. Use this information to identify patterns and make informed decisions about your lifestyle and treatment.

2. **Understanding Results:**
   - Familiarize yourself with your target blood sugar ranges and interpret your results accordingly. Recognize the significance of fasting and postprandial readings in maintaining optimal glucose control during pregnancy.

3. **Adaptation and Adjustment:**
   - Embrace the need for adaptation and adjustment. Your healthcare team may recommend modifications to your diet, exercise routine, or medication based on your individual response to treatment and changing needs throughout pregnancy.

4. **Healthy Lifestyle Choices:**

- Prioritize a healthy lifestyle, incorporating balanced nutrition, regular physical activity, and stress management. These choices contribute not only to blood sugar control but also to your overall well-being.

5. **Effective Communication:**
   - Maintain open and effective communication with your healthcare team. Share your concerns, ask questions, and actively participate in discussions about your gestational diabetes management plan.

6. **Positive Mindset:**
   - Approach the management of gestational diabetes with a positive mindset. Celebrate successes, no matter how small, and view challenges as opportunities for learning and improvement.

7. **Individualized Approach:**
   - Recognize that gestational diabetes management is highly individualized. Your healthcare team considers factors unique to your health, pregnancy, and lifestyle when tailoring recommendations and setting targets.

8. **Embracing Support:**
   - Seek support from your loved ones, friends, and healthcare providers. A supportive network can play a crucial role in helping you navigate the challenges associated with gestational diabetes.

9. **Preparation for Postpartum:**
   - Consider the potential impact of gestational diabetes on postpartum health. Continue healthy habits beyond pregnancy, and discuss long-term lifestyle strategies with your healthcare team.

10. **Anticipating Changes:**
   - Be prepared for changes in your management plan as your pregnancy progresses. Regular reassessment and adjustments ensure that your plan aligns with your evolving needs.

Remember, managing gestational diabetes is a collaborative effort between you and your healthcare team. By actively participating in your care, staying informed, and maintaining a positive approach, you can navigate this journey successfully. The ultimate goal is to promote the health and well-being of both you and your baby, laying the foundation for a positive pregnancy experience and a healthy start to parenthood.

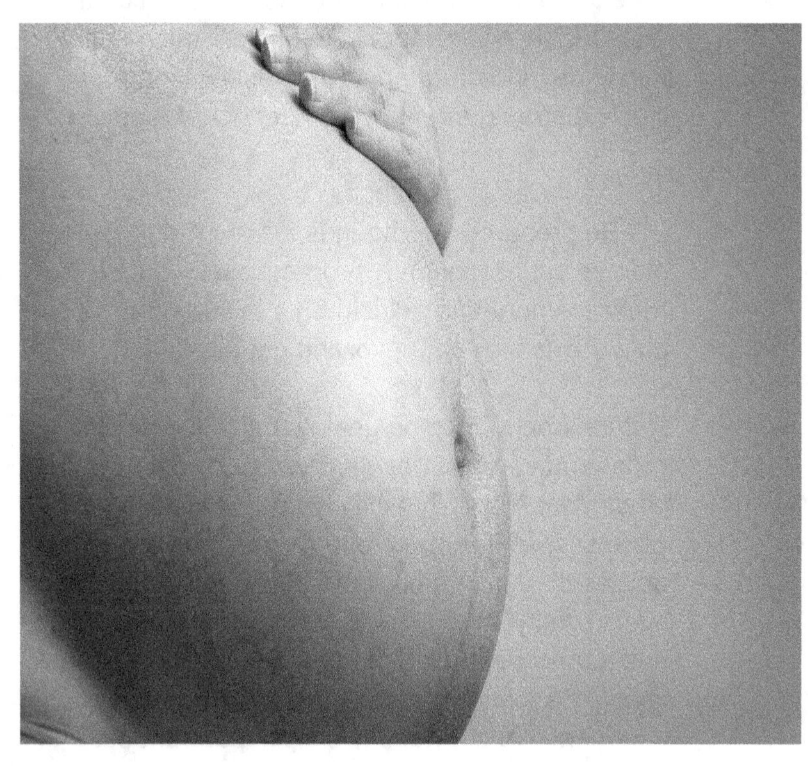

www.ingramcontent.com/pod-product-compliance
Lightning Source LLC
Chambersburg PA
CBHW070824260726
48660CB00005B/1982